# Thinking Thin Through Spiritual and Mental Steps

A Companion Guide to Help You Succeed on Your Journey to Healthy and Permanent Weight Loss

## Dr. Pamela S. Chapman

Copyright © 2014 by Dr. Pamela S. Chapman

All Rights Reserved

The reader is allowed to copy all worksheets that may be helpful for personal use. All other aspects of this book, in whole or part, including the right of reproduction, are reserved by the author.

No other part of this book may be used or reproduced by any means, graphic, electronic, or mechanical, including photocopying, scanning, recording, or by any information storage retrieval system, without the express written permission of the author, except in the case of brief quotations in articles or reviews.

This book is designed to provide information and motivation to readers. No warranties or guarantees are expressed or implied by the inclusion of any material or exercises in this book. It is sold with the understanding that neither the author or publisher are engaged to render any type of psychological, legal, or any other kind of professional advice. The information provided in this book is designed solely to provide helpful information on the subjects discussed. This book is not meant to be used to diagnose or treat any medical or psychological condition. For diagnosis or treatment of any medical or psychological issue, consult an appropriately licensed professional practitioner. The publisher and author are neither responsible, nor liable for any damages or negative consequences to any person reading or acting upon the information in this book. As a reader, you are responsible for your own choices, actions, and results. References are provided for informational purposes only and do not constitute endorsement of any websites or other sources. Readers should be aware that web links listed in this book may change.

Published by:
Empower People Ventures
PO Box 179098
San Diego, CA 92117

ISBN: 978-0-9895452-4-2
Produced in the United States of America

Library of Congress Control Number: 2014952870

First Printing, 2014

## DEDICATION

This book is dedicated to my beloved husband John. You have taught me so much about self-acceptance, love and patience. Your love, support and endless belief in me are my greatest joys! And to my sister, Anita Hajos; your love and encouragement have been a constant source of inspiration and strength throughout my life. You walk a path of peace and faith as a role model of sanity for me now and during our turbulent youth. I will always be grateful!

I thank God for the presence of both of you in my life. You are the wind beneath my wings.

*"The first wealth is health."*

Ralph Waldo Emerson

# Table of Contents

How to Get the Most Out of This Book ........................................................... 1

Introduction .................................................................................................... 3

Chapter One: The Challenge and the Answer ................................................ 5

    My Commitment to Thinking Thin and Healthy ....................................... 11

Chapter Two: Self-Image ............................................................................. 15

    Two Images Worksheet ............................................................................ 21

Chapter Three: Prayer .................................................................................. 25

    The Teachings of Jesus ............................................................................ 26

    Prayer Treatment for Health and Ideal Weight ........................................ 30

    My Prayer Treatment for Health and Ideal Weight ................................. 31

Chapter Four: Your Feelings ........................................................................ 35

    Feeling My Feelings Worksheet .............................................................. 41

    Changing My Feelings ............................................................................. 44

    Changing My Feelings Worksheet ........................................................... 45

Chapter Five: What You Focus On .............................................................. 49

    Things I Love About My Body Worksheet ............................................. 53

    What I Want Worksheet .......................................................................... 55

    My Joy Journal ........................................................................................ 59

Chapter Six: Change .................................................................................... 63

    My Physical State Worksheet .................................................................. 67

    Cost/Benefit Worksheet ........................................................................... 71

    My Dozen Alternative Behaviors List ..................................................... 73

Chapter Seven: Are You Smushed? ............................................................. 77

    The Obituary for: .................................................................................... 79

    My Accomplishments .............................................................................. 81

    Goals I Want to Accomplish ................................................................... 85

    My Personal Time Schedule .................................................................... 89

What's Next? ................................................................................................ 95

Acknowledgements .................................................................................... 101

About the Author ....................................................................................... 103

End Notes ................................................................................................... 105

*"He who mounts a wild elephant goes where the wild elephant goes!"*

Randolph Bournes

# How to Get the Most Out of This Book

Thank you for investing in this print version of *Thinking Thin through Spiritual and Mental Steps*. I want to acknowledge that this has been designed as a workbook – as the subtitle says, it's *"A Companion Guide to Help You Succeed on Your Journey to Healthy and Permanent Weight Loss."* This companion guide contains several worksheets, which you will want to use in order to get the full value out of the information and exercises contained herein.

No matter what diet or exercise program you are currently following this guidebook is designed to help you enhance your self-esteem and body image. Each chapter includes exercises and worksheets that will add depth and understanding to the material presented. Completing them can make losing weight and maintaining that weight loss a more joyful experience.

Knowing information can be helpful; truly understanding it can be transformational. Therefore, to obtain the greatest value from this workbook, allow yourself plenty of time to read the material and set aside 15-20 minutes to complete each worksheet. To get the most value from the visualization exercises, plan on 5-10 minutes of uninterrupted time in a quiet and private space. Allow yourself time to take a few deep breaths, close your eyes, fully relax your body and to experience your ideal self, using all your senses. Imagine the scene as though it is actually occurring in that moment. Visualizing yourself as trim, fit and making healthy choices can help enormously in developing your new slimmer and healthier self-image.

The journey toward your healthy weight can be a time filled with opportunities to adjust your self perception and truly learn to love yourself. I hope that you will embrace this opportunity!

Here's to your health and happiness!

Dr. Pam

*"A year from now you will wish you had started today."*

Karen Lamb

# Introduction

The media is filled with reminders of the worldwide epidemic of obesity and diabetes. The statistics are astounding: *more than one third of adults and seventeen percent of youth in the United States are obese*[i]. Also, this figure represents a three to seven year lifespan loss for these individuals and dramatically increased chances for developing hypertension, heart disease, diabetes and arthritis. The problem seems to be spiraling out of control with forecasts *doubling* the storm of obesity in the next 20 years! The problem persists even with the finest of diets, exercise programs and increasing awareness all in place. Why is this happening?

This is not just another diet book. I believe that nutritional knowledge and portion control are absolutely necessary for lifelong weight management and maintenance. However, if portion control were the total answer, this entire epidemic would have been solved a long time ago. I see the obesity epidemic as a natural response to the crazy stresses and over-frenzied pace of our current lifestyles. The over-consumption of food has become the answer for millions of people who are seeking satisfaction and not finding it in their everyday existence.

All foods, when broken down to their chemical components, are powerful means of altering brain chemistry. For example, we've all experienced stimulation after eating chocolate and relaxation after eating a turkey dinner. Everything you eat contributes to your mood and energy. The food choices you make alter your chemical balance, which then affects your lifestyle and ongoing food choices.

Our brains are wired for survival and finding satisfaction is a large part of this process. You will note the foods you tend to seek are not fruits and vegetables, but are highly processed, high sugar, high fat treats that thrill the taste buds and change your mood. The search for emotional satisfaction can lead you to the corner grocery store or straight to your refrigerator. This book will help you identify healthy, alternative ways to decrease stress and break emotional eating habits. My goal in writing this book is to help you get to your healthy weight and to eliminate the blame and guilt you may feel about your body and eating habits. I will help you see that your struggle with weight and over-eating is a response to stress, depression and/or poor self-esteem. *If you choose, you can find another answer that will bring you happiness and improve your health at the same time.*

*There is definitely a way out of this "diet-and-binge" pattern and there is a way to end the roller coaster of emotions that is so often the cause of over-eating.* This book includes several powerful ideas and worksheets, which will map out your personal path to healthy weight and improved self-esteem.

*"Tell me what you eat, and I will tell you who you are."*

Briallat-Savarin

# Chapter One: The Challenge and the Answer

I am excited to share some ideas on the importance of mental outlook and attitude on weight loss, improved health and the overall well-being of your body. The information I'll be sharing with you has come from my own personal experience with weight loss and my 25 years of experience as a psychotherapist.

First of all, I'm sure it is obvious that our society has become obsessed with weight loss and diets. We are a nation obsessed with thinness. Hollywood and the fashion industry hold up an image of pencil-thin women – actually underweight by health standards – as the desired goal. The severe measures of diet and exercise that these women follow are unrealistic for the typical person to attempt. Society's idolization of the unrealistic norm sets up a perfect breeding ground for self-loathing and general bad feelings about our bodies.

Studies show that over 67% of Americans are overweight (and/or obese) and the enormous health implications related to being overweight are staggering. *Over 70 million Americans suffer from insulin resistance and are encountering metabolic syndrome.* Metabolic syndrome is a precursor to diabetes[ii]. The amazing fact is that this epidemic is developing at a time when more is known about the prevention and treatment of obesity and diabetes than at any time in history. In fact, Americans spend over 50 billion dollars a year on weight loss aids sold through doctors or over the counter, yet only 10% of dieters succeed at their weight loss goals. Of those 10% of successful dieters, only 20% maintain their weight loss over the long term[iii]. *These statistics prove that an important piece is missing from our current diet mentality. I believe the most important missing piece is the mental/spiritual link.*

As humans, we are mind/body beings. We create through the efforts of our bodies and the use of our minds. We are taught that when we decide to lose weight and begin a weight loss program, we must change our eating habits and/or change our exercise habits, yet few people learn to focus on changing their mental habits as well. An essential aspect of achieving lasting weight loss is the mental/spiritual work that needs to be included in any successful weight reduction program.

It is known in psychology, religion, and sports psychology that how you *think* and what you *feel* are essential in achieving your desired outcomes in life. Cognitive therapy teaches that what you think about, what you say to yourself and what your core beliefs are about situations in your life are more important to mood outcome than the circumstances you encounter. Religion teaches us that as you believe in your heart, so shall it be in your life. "As you believe in your heart" refers to your feelings. This includes emotion and your mental image of yourself. Sports psychology teaches to visualize your success, to actually feel the experience; the successful swing of the golf club or tennis racket, and see in your mind the perfect placement of the ball. The mental image and the feeling attached to it increase the likelihood of improvement in the sport.

In these examples the focus is on the goal or the desired outcome. When you focus on what you want, feel the outcome in your heart, and have an expectation of that desired outcome occurring, the likelihood of your desired outcome is significantly increased. In fact, it is nearly guaranteed. The world's current philosophy of dieting puts you in a position of automatically focusing on what you don't want. Diets usually start because you feel terrible about yourself; you've reached the end of your rope and have limited positive feelings about your body. The emphasis is on what you *don't* want: being overweight, or feeling out of control or shameful about your body. *Seldom is the emphasis on what you do want: the vision of yourself as slender, energetic and in perfect health. What would happen if you changed the emphasis to focus on what you do want?*

The key is to remember that whatever you say to yourself on an ongoing basis becomes your future reality. It doesn't happen by magic, but by a known mental/spiritual function. The things you consciously say or think to yourself over and over eventually become subconscious belief systems. Once a thought becomes a subconscious belief, it tends to become habit and easily brings forth similar results in your life. Another way you can consciously communicate with your subconscious mind is through images—through visualizing your desired outcome.

Visualization is a powerful technique that has long been used by athletes. Tiger Woods is a perfect example of this behavior. He hesitates before swinging a golf club—you can actually see him take the few extra seconds to do this before he swings the club. What he's doing is visualizing a perfect swing. He's feeling the club make exactly the right contact with the ball and seeing the ball land exactly where he wants it to go. If Tiger Woods started his swing feeling unfit, terrible about himself and doubting his success, the end result would be very different.

*Thinking Thin Through Spiritual and Mental Steps*

*How do you typically set yourself up mentally to diet? Is it for success or failure?* Developing a mental visualization, a clear picture of the desired body size and shape you want is essential to achieving your desired outcome. If the mental picture you hold of yourself is one of being overweight, making poor food choices and feeling out of control, then even following the best diet and exercise plan in the world will not be successful.

In my days of dieting prior to realizing the importance of the mental step, there were many times when I went on a diet, lost ten pounds with great effort and struggle, then quickly regained fifteen pounds with the greatest of ease! It's no wonder that we can feel so helpless in our dieting attempts when even valiant efforts result in failure. So, what's the way out? How can you stop the diet insanity? How can you live a healthy and active life without carrying excess weight that hampers your quality of life and at times causes horrific health consequences? Living in health and balance is the way your life is meant to flow. It is possible to regain the self-acceptance and positive body image you naturally deserve. You can do this with ease and joy by consciously and subconsciously making choices that contribute to your health and ideal weight.

Let's start with a brief description of how the mind works, and then move on to ways that your mind can support your diet efforts. The mind is divided into two functions – the conscious and the subconscious. Each serves in different capacities. The conscious mind makes evaluations based on your five senses and you make conscious choices based on the data you've obtained. You reason and think with your conscious mind. The subconscious mind controls your body's automatic functions such as heartbeat and breathing. It also develops habits to simplify your life. For example, have you ever settled into the driver's seat of your car and the next thing you knew, you were at your destination? Or, did you have to think about how to tie your shoes this morning? Can you imagine how difficult each day would be if you had to consciously make choices about how to tie your shoes, start the car or brush your teeth? Your subconscious mind actually liberates you from the task of making these decisions. These routine tasks take effort at first, but gradually they go from the conscious to the subconscious mind and liberate you from having to choose each mundane detail.

The subconscious mind has no filtering ability; it doesn't know the difference between healthy and unhealthy, truth and error. Whatever you consciously say or do repeatedly, filters into the subconscious mind and becomes a habit. Eating is an action that you need to do repeatedly for survival. If you are overweight your habitual patterns are likely leading you to make automatic choices, *subconscious* choices, that don't support your desire of being at your ideal weight. How many times have you found yourself eating something without even thinking about it?

Here's an example of how this occurs: When I was much younger, I made the extremely important discovery that when I got stressed or upset, eating pastry or candy – actually any processed carbohydrate – would relax me and bring me back to my desired, calmer mood. We lived near a bakery and I always had a ready supply of delicious choices. As time went on, the awareness of this calming technique slipped into my subconscious mind and if I experienced any negative emotion, I automatically reached for my carbohydrate fix. It was a solution that didn't ultimately support me, and my weight ballooned to 228 pounds. The amazing thing is, I was rarely making conscious food choices. I was more like a pre-programmed robot responding to circumstances in my life. My subconscious mind, in an attempt to simplify and improve my life, led me to choices that actually harmed my body. After a multitude of unsuccessful or only partially successful dieting attempts, it became clear to me that both my habits and my body image needed to change in order to support my weight loss efforts. I started to learn about the subconscious mind and realized the power it had in my habits and lifestyle. It was at this point that I began to have dramatic success with my food choices.

Earlier I mentioned that as you believe in your heart, so shall your life be. The heart refers to a state of feeling and the subconscious mind is the powerhouse of emotions and automatic reactions. It can be a friend or foe in your dieting efforts. In order to *be* thin, you must be able to *feel* thin and *see* yourself thin in mind. This is not an easy task when you're dieting, given that you are most likely feeling fat and out of control. So, how can you feel thin when you're not? How can you feel in control when your experience has been that you're out of control? There is an answer!

Your trusted friend, the subconscious mind, comes into play here. Another amazing feature of the subconscious mind is that it has no ability to tell the difference between an actual situation and one that has been actively imagined. It will take both situations from the conscious mind and store them in the subconscious mind as experiences that have actually occurred. The more you give yourself the consciously imagined experience, the more quickly the message will filter into the subconscious mind and support a new, healthy habit – one that will support you in the direction of your desire. As your subconscious mind gets the clear picture of you at your ideal weight, you will find yourself easily making conscious choices that support your vision of a slimmer self.

Of important note – the subconscious mind is also referred to as the *subjective* mind because it is subject to the *conscious* mind. You have conscious control of what goes into your subconscious mind by what you consciously choose to place your attention and thoughts on. This is important to realize because what goes into your subconscious mind becomes the thought patterns and habits you develop. *You can think of this change of mentality as a cleansing process.* If you view your negative habits and self-destructive thoughts as dirty water in a glass and imagine your new, positive visualizations and statements as clean water flowing into the glass, you can see that over time the clean water will replace the dirty water.

## **Notes/Journaling**

___
___
___
___
___
___
___
___
___
___
___
___
___
___
___
___
___
___
___

# Tools

There are several ways you can consciously cause subconscious changes to come about. The remainder of this book will be a detailed explanation of a variety of different tools. *These tools include prayer/treatment, visualization, and journaling exercises that will help you reach your weight and health goals with greater ease while increasing the likelihood of permanent change.* We will also explore the effects of certain brain chemicals, serotonin, endorphin and dopamine in particular, on mood and appetite

On the next page, you'll find a worksheet titled *"My Commitment to Thinking Thin and Healthy."* Using this worksheet to track your progress will enable you to develop new behaviors. Date the steps as you begin each process. I believe that with these tools you can join the ranks of successful dieters who achieve ultimate victory in the search for lifelong ideal weight.

# Notes/Journaling

_____
_____
_____
_____
_____
_____
_____
_____
_____
_____
_____
_____
_____

*Thinking Thin Through Spiritual and Mental Steps*

# My Commitment to Thinking Thin and Healthy

START DATE: _____

Visualize yourself thin for five to ten minutes every day. (**Two Images,** Ch. 2)   _____

Write an affirmation, prayer or treatment that encompasses all areas of your perfect health and review daily.
(**My Prayer Treatment for Health and Ideal Weight,** Ch. 3)   _____

Practice **Feeling My Feelings** (hunger, anger, exhaustion, etc.) versus thoughts (I'm bored, it's time to eat, etc,).
(**Feeling My Feelings**, Ch. 4)   _____

Complete a **Changing My Feelings** Journal entry daily.
(**Changing My Feelings,** Ch. 4)   _____

Journal **Three Things I Love About My Body** every day.
(**Three Things I Love About My Body,** Ch. 5)   _____

Work on the **What I Want** exercise daily. (**What I Want,** Ch. 5)   _____

Choose one activity daily to increase your serotonin (calming) and/or increase your endorphin (pleasure) levels. (**Serotonin and Endorphin,** Ch. 5)   _____

Write daily in **My Joy Journal** three things that make you happy.
(**My Joy Journal**, Ch. 5)   _____

Complete **My Physical State** worksheet, **Cost Benefit** and
**My Dozen Alternative Behaviors List** worksheets.
(All 3 worksheets, Ch. 6)   _____

Complete and review **The Obituary Of, My Accomplishments,**
**Goals I Want to Accomplish,** and **Personal Time Schedule**. Review often to ensure your daily tasks correspond with your goals and desires.
(All 4 worksheets, Ch. 7)   _____

# Notes/Journaling

## Notes/Journaling

*"Nobody can go back and start a new beginning, but anyone can start today and make a new ending."*

Maria Robinson

# Chapter Two: Self-Image

In this chapter, I will share with you how self-image develops and the critical nature of self-image with regard to weight loss and maintaining a healthy lifestyle. *We'll look at self-image through the eyes of psychology and will explore ways you can alter your self-image naturally and easily.*

You have a unique, personally developed picture of yourself that you hold in your mind. This image is referred to as your self-image. Self-image is created over time by your repetitive thoughts and beliefs about your body and abilities along with exposure to images and the messages you get from people you trust. This foolishly includes the media. You actually form a mental picture, an idea of yourself and also an idea of what is ideal.

Unfortunately eight out of ten women are dissatisfied with their appearance[iv]. Most women engage in negative self-talk and ultimately suffer from poor self-image. If you are like most women these disempowering thoughts about yourself become the core beliefs from which you build your actions and your lifestyle. Poor self-image comes mostly from comparing yourself to your mental picture of the "ideal" and then making a judgment about yourself based on that comparison. When you compare your body to the airbrushed, computer-enhanced models you see in magazines and on television, you are given an opportunity to evaluate yourself as imperfect. Once your subconscious mind buys into this belief system, you judge all of your life experiences through this filter and become convinced there is something wrong with you. The reality is, there is nothing wrong with you! *You are only a new thought away from being your ideal, healthy self.*

How you feel, your mood and your acceptance or lack of acceptance of yourself is based more on what you say to yourself than on the actual experiences in your life. *Your words, silently spoken to yourself, alter your brain chemistry and your mood in seconds.* Through your thoughts and words, you can speak yourself into anxiety and overeating, or you can calm yourself with words, thoughts and images that bring you back into your body and center you in the moment.

What you consciously choose to say to yourself or think about over time filters to the subconscious level of your mind. This impacts first your self-image, then your behavior and ultimately what you end up experiencing in your life. All of life is experienced in your mind. It is there you experience all the events of your life and assign value to them. All you experience in your outer world, the material world, was first a thought in mind. As your thoughts become beliefs they become part of your subconscious, and from this position, they begin to color the experiences of your life.

Once these thoughts are accepted by your subconscious mind, they automatically affect your mood, actually producing changes in your body chemistry that affect your emotions, hunger, desires and image of yourself. You can, through inaccurate thinking, develop a self-image that is totally in error and thus experience in your mind a life that doesn't support your highest potential. *The opposite is also true. You can, through definite use of your mind, develop a picture of yourself that can bring you great joy and satisfaction.*

The most dramatic example I can think of to highlight the inaccuracies of a negative self-image occurred during a conversation I had many years ago. It was one of those learning moments that altered me forever.

I was completing my Master's Degree in Social Work and working at a hospital. I learned that there was a woman, a few years my junior, who was an intern in the Psychology Department, and just a few months away from completing her Ph.D. I was stunned to learn she had been in the Olympics and won a bronze medal. I was totally in awe! First of all, I was so proud of myself for being just a few months away from my Master's and here she was, younger than I, finishing her Ph.D.! I was so proud of her – and then to learn she had won a bronze medal in an international competition! I was determined to get to know her.

I joined her for lunch, and gushed my admiration and awe. I asked her what plans she had to celebrate the momentous occasion of her doctorate. She replied, in all seriousness and with little expression, that her graduation really wasn't cause for celebration because she'd struggled with her thesis and was actually graduating a couple of years later than her friends, which caused her some embarrassment. I decided I'd switch the topic – no fun talking about school with her – so we turned to sports. I shared with her (again gushing my admiration) that I'd just learned she had won a medal at the Olympics. This is truly an amazing accomplishment on anyone's list of credentials and I knew she would have amazing stories and emotions to share.

Well, she did… have emotions that amazed me, that is. She remarked how embarrassing it was to win a bronze medal! She believed she deserved to win the gold and would be disappointed for the rest of her life at her terrible performance that day!

I was dumbstruck! Here I was sitting with a beautiful, brilliant young woman – a woman beginning her adult life with experiences and successes that very few people would accomplish in a lifetime – and *all she saw was her lack*. It was, and still is, the most vivid example I've experienced of poor self-image impacting one's experience of self. Her life experience, and her mental experience of it were not on the same page or even in the same book! Her repetitious, self-defeating statements about not being #1 or perfect had settled into her subconscious mind and now everything was filtered through these gray glasses. Like all of us, she carried a mental picture of herself and she carried on a continuous conversation with herself that interpreted every situation she encountered. She could have changed her thoughts and been in celebration of all she accomplished. You can change your thinking and self-image and in the process change your life!

*Within you there is the power and the intelligence to make any change you want in your life.* You can call upon this intelligence through the power of your subconscious mind to change your body image, your prosperity image, and actually, any image of yourself that you desire. A famous quote of 20th century philosopher Ernest Holmes is "Change your thinking, change your life."

Let's look at the process of changing your thinking. Research on hypnosis proved that *the fastest means of changing thought is to imagine yourself exactly as you desire to be while you are in a relaxed state.* There is no effort or will power utilized in making the change. All beliefs and habits, including your eating habits, are made in the same relaxed way. Changing your beliefs must happen in a relaxed environment, one that is easy and free of will power, discipline or denial. When you focus on the use of will power, you are actually looking at lack and living in an antagonistic experience of the changes you desire to make. Attempting to use effort or will power puts your actions (which you're forcing) into immediate conflict with your mental image (the picture of yourself). When your actions and your mental image are in conflict, your mental image (which is subconscious) always wins. Let's examine how that conflict occurs. As we discussed earlier, we all have one mind that is divided into two distinct functions:

## The Conscious vs. the Unconscious Minds

| The Conscious | The Unconscious |
|---|---|
| • Makes choices. | • Works automatically. |
| • Draws conclusions. | • Includes self-image. |
| • Gathers information. | • Automatically maintains body functions…breathing, heart pumping, cell repairing. |
| • Evaluates data. | • Takes thoughts from the conscious and accepts them as true. |
| • Compares. | • Implements without question. |
| • Makes observations. | • Stores information through repetition and belief. |
| • Judges. | • Is the storehouse of all knowledge. |
| • Initiates action through making choices. "I choose…" is a conscious decision. | • It knows how to automatically put into action what is required to accomplish your desires. |
| • The conscious mind cannot create results. | |

Information in the subconscious mind is stored through repetition and belief. The subconscious mind holds the self-image and works effortlessly to maintain the self-image you have. If your subconscious mind has a picture of you being heavier than you wish to be, even if you achieve your ideal weight by dieting, your subconscious mind will automatically find every means to bring your weight back to your original self-image if your self-image hasn't changed. As a psychotherapy student, I learned the best way to identify a person's self-talk or self-image was to look at the reality of circumstances in their life. Your thought, once believed, always manifests! It has no option but to do so. Once information is believed, it filters to the subconscious mind where it is automatically brought into form. If you are overweight, it is guaranteed that your mental picture of yourself is overweight. If you are plagued by a health problem, or a habit that doesn't support your health, it is guaranteed you have a mental picture of yourself that corresponds with this behavior. Let me use myself as an example. This is amazing in its simplicity and its uncanny manifestation in my life.

When I was a young child the things I wanted most were love, a sense of belonging and safety – the same things all children long for. The world I learned from consisted of my family, school and friends. The one person I knew who "had it all" was a family friend: Mrs. K. Whether Mrs. K. actually "had it all" or not is beside the point. The point is that I *thought* she did. The experience I had in mind was the most important thing – it was this that became stored in my subconscious mind and then the universe found the means to make it my reality.

Mrs. K. had a handsome husband who genuinely adored her. They were successful business owners and they demonstrated an unquestionable mutual respect. Mrs. K. was attractive and she also happened to be at least eighty pounds overweight. She visited us often and whenever she left, I always told my Mother and sister, "When I grow up I want to be *exactly* like Mrs. K." My family would laugh at my infatuation, because the primary feature that they thought of with Mrs. K. was her obesity. Coming from a family of abuse that struggled financially, the experience in my mind was of her perfection. What I meant was that I wanted joy, a rewarding business, and a successful relationship. But I continued to say, "I want to be *exactly* like Mrs. K." As I became an adult the out-picturing of my life became very similar to Mrs. K.'s, including the successful business, the handsome, loving husband...*and* the eighty pounds of excess weight.

**Two facts to remember:**

1. Your actions and behavior are *always* consistent with your self-image. For example: my image of being "*exactly* like Mrs. K." demonstrated in my life".

2. The self-image can *always* be consciously changed and it can include all the positive aspects of what you want. I could have consciously chosen to be loved and successful like Mrs. K. and chosen to be thin instead of stating, "I want to be *exactly* like Mrs. K."

We are not talking about positive thinking, because positive thinking, which is a conscious activity, doesn't work if it is in conflict with your subconscious self-image. Remember this premise: when your actions are in conflict with your mental image, your mental image (the subconscious picture of self) always wins. For example, if your self-image is that you are overweight, you may be able to control your food intake for a limited amount of time and lose weight. However, you can anticipate a return to your original overweight status unless you change your self-image along the way. Your self-image and your habits go hand in hand. You must change your self-image in order for your habits to change. So, let's get to work on the creation of a new self-image for you, one that supports your desired vision of perfect health, vitality and happiness!

To start, you will actively visualize being at your ideal weight, living in a healthy manner and making food choices that support your newly found mental slimness. Following the exercise, you will have a clear picture of your goal self. Write on the "**Two Images**" worksheet (located on the next page) what you looked like and what you felt like being thin and living thin during this exercise. Remember, research has shown that the fastest way to change your self-image is to imagine yourself exactly as you desire to be and to do so while in a relaxed state. So let's have you relax and start imagining!

Sit comfortably, take a deep breath and exhale. Then another. Breathe in calm, safe, peaceful energy and breathe out the stress and strain of the day. Continue to breathe deeply, filling your stomach with cleansing air, and exhaling fully. Once you are fully relaxed, see yourself at your ideal weight, dressed in a flattering outfit, standing before a mirror. Notice how your body looks, notice the contours of your torso, the firm shape of your arms and legs. Notice the attractive and slender shape of your face. Take a couple of minutes to truly notice the details of your healthy and beautiful body. Next, notice how you feel. Notice the pride and joy you experience in recognizing how healthy and trim your body is. Notice how energetic and fit you feel. Fully experience how wonderful you look and feel.

Next, imagine yourself at a small gathering of friends. Notice yourself looking fit and attractive. See yourself enjoying the company of your friends. Notice your focus is on the pleasure of friendship and you feel 100% comfortable in this situation. Now, see yourself making healthy food choices, naturally choosing foods you know support your health and appearance. Feel good about your choices. Feel the pleasure and pride you experience in being a naturally thin eater. After you have visualized yourself in both scenes, take a few minutes to write down the experience – what did you look like? How did you feel? On the following page, write down the details. Remember to focus on the feeling: how it feels being healthy, attractive and in control.

*Thinking Thin Through Spiritual and Mental Steps*
## Two Images Worksheet

1. <u>**You in the mirror,**</u> **attractively attired and in perfect shape at your healthiest weight.**

   _____
   _____
   _____
   _____
   _____
   _____
   _____
   _____

2. <u>**You at a party,**</u> **enjoying yourself and making healthy food choices.**

   _____
   _____
   _____
   _____
   _____
   _____
   _____
   _____

In order to help these images become part of your subconscious, and assist you in your goal of achieving ideal body weight, spend 5 to 10 minutes each morning or evening imagining both scenes. Pick the time that works best for you and **do it consistently.** Turn to "**My Commitment to Thinking Thin and Healthy**" and mark the date you commit to this daily practice.

# Notes/Journaling

# Notes/Journaling

*"Your vision is the promise of what you shall one day be; your ideal is the prophecy of what you shall at last unveil."*

James Allen

# Chapter Three: Prayer

I can think of no greater tool than prayer for creating changes in your physical health and body weight. This chapter will cover how to write a prayer and discuss some of the teachings of Jesus that pertain to prayer. People have used prayer for thousands of years to find answers to mankind's problems. When you use prayer, it is imperative that you pray with the full answer in mind. When you begin in full expectation, having faith that the desired outcome as seen in your mind must appear, your prayers are answered. According to the Bible, Jesus told us to pray believing it has already been done unto you. The teachings of Jesus reveal to us that there is a law, which responds to your thoughts. The extent to which your prayers are answered depends upon your faith. If you pray with doubt, without belief or faith, the result will be a lack of manifestation.

You are a spiritual being who is on a human journey. Your job is to discover what you want, what your good is and allow that good to flow to you as a gift of grace. The good comes to you not from conscious effort, but from your thoughts infused with faith and feeling. Your prayers, when uttered without feeling, and certainly without faith, are likely to miss the mark of manifestation. Your prayers need to be stated in joyful expectancy and excitement, with absolute belief and faith. When stated in this way, prayers attract more and more good to you.

Knowing that prayer always works and that it responds to your faith, isn't it odd that we try to "attack" the problem of overweight and obesity with diets and exercise versus prayer? Let's see what Jesus had to say about thinking, prayer and faith with regard to physical health and a perfect body. You'll note He makes no reference to whether high carbohydrate or high protein diets work best! There is room for your reflections and thoughts under each of the sayings of Jesus.

# The Teachings of Jesus

**Matthew 7:7 – "Ask and it will be given you, search and you will find."**

    If you turn over your need to control your eating and your weight to the Higher Power within you, you will find the way…the right answer to becoming naturally thin and healthy

**Mark 9:23 – "If you can believe, all things are possible to one who believes."**

    Believe in yourself and in the Spirit of God within you. You must first believe, and when you do, you will be in control of the food you eat and your attitudes about yourself!

**Mark 10:52 – "Go on your way. Your faith has made you whole."**

    Trust in God to direct the thoughts you have about food. As you learn to trust, you will eat naturally those foods which bless your body.

**Mark 11:24 – "What soever things ye desire, pray as if ye had already received them, and ye shall have them."**

    Pray with a grateful heart, *knowing* and *feeling* beyond a shadow of a doubt that God will hear you and respond!

**Mark 12:29 – "Love yourself."**

This says it all. Love yourself just as you are, right now, in this moment. As you truly express love to yourself, you will naturally come to use food as a tool to embrace life, not to sabotage your dream.

**Luke 8:48 – "Be at ease. Your faith has made you whole; go in peace."**

Release your fears that you must be in control. When you are trusting, you can let go and feel peaceful about your body and the food you eat.

**Luke 12:29 – "Don't worry about what you shall eat or what you shall drink. Do not doubt. Your Father knows what you need."**

You can trust the process of food nourishing your body; it is not an enemy. Trust in God's direction. He knows exactly what you need to balance the process of food intake in your body temple.

**John 5:5 – "Will you choose to be made whole?"**

Always, you must *choose* to unite your thinking with the wisdom and intelligence of Infinite Mind. When you make this choice, there is nothing, absolutely nothing, that can keep you from realizing your desire!

**John 5:8 – "Rise, take up your burden and walk."**

    Rise to the level of understanding that you are in charge with the infinite assistance of God. Make your decision, and take charge of your life. You <u>can</u> do it with the power of God within you!

**John 7:24 – "Judge not by appearances, but judge with right thinking."**

    Don't judge yourself by someone else's opinion. Judge what is right for <u>your</u> body. Your body was never meant to be the image of thinness you see portrayed in the media today as the "perfect body." Judge yourself with wisdom…right thinking!

**James 1:5 – "If any of you lacks wisdom, he should ask God, who gives generously to all without finding fault, and it will be given to him."**

    God does not judge you or fault you. Ask for the knowledge and support that you need, and it will be given to you. You can, with greater ease, make changes in your body image and habits when you ask God for help!

Have you ever wondered why some prayers are answered and others are not? It is the Father's *good pleasure* to fulfill all your desires and we know that God does not have favorites. *The Isaiah Effect*, by Gregg Braden, is my favorite book about prayer. He emphasizes the importance of *feeling* in your prayers. As you pray it is important to do so in full expectation of the answer and to experience the emotions you would experience as if your prayers were already answered. He actually points out that prayers of petition, or *prayers of asking, are frequently ineffective because the focus of thought and feeling is on your lack instead of your desired outcome*[v].

To give thanks for all that you already have and to express gratitude in advance while knowing your desired outcome is on its way is the greatest form of faith – as is the exercise of feeling the request manifested. Jesus always said *"Thank you, Father," knowing in advance that His prayers were answered.* It is to acknowledge with absolute certainty the power of God.

You will notice in the following chapters many opportunities to practice feeling your desired outcome. Feeling sends a loud and clear message to the subconscious mind, which stores a visualized scene that is imagined (with feeling) as a memory, *as if the incident actually took place.* When you use prayer, make sure you deny everything in mind that does not convey your desired outcome. Do this while you pray and also later as you walk through your day. Keep your eyes on the desired outcome, not on the speed bumps on the road. As you walk through your day, with your gaze on your goal, recognize it as a certainty. Note everything big and small that demonstrates it is coming toward you. It will help erase doubt by returning your mind to seeing the complete out-picturing of your desire.

Recognizing that your faith, your belief and your mental equivalent are the keys to the physical forms in your life, let's look at an example of an affirmative prayer treatment for perfect health and body shape. Remember to pray with great feeling. *Saying the words and not feeling them in your heart will <u>not</u> lead to the desired outcome.*

(Example)
## Prayer Treatment for Health and Ideal Weight

I know there is one God. God is the presence, power and intelligence in all, through all, in the seen and unseen world. I know God is all beauty, health and wisdom. God is all knowledge and perfect understanding. There being only One God, One Presence, from which all is made, I know I am one with God... the God source flows through me as me. I am one with the ever-present power, health and intelligence of God.

I know the wisdom, health and beauty of God are one with my life now. I know that each choice I make naturally moves me toward perfect health. I focus on the truth of my being and recognize that I am one with God. All that is the Father's is mine now in this moment to enjoy. I believe it is the will of God for me to live in absolute health and at my ideal weight. I joyously accept God's goodness and health. I give great thanks for all the abundance of life, health and happiness, which are now mine.

Amen


Now, practice writing an affirmation, prayer or treatment that encompasses all areas of your perfect health. Read your prayer daily and record the date of your commitment on "**My Commitment to Thinking Thin and Healthy.**"

*Thinking Thin Through Spiritual and Mental Steps*

**My Prayer Treatment for Health and Ideal Weight**

# Notes/Journaling

# Notes/Journaling

*"You are living in integrity when the life you are living on the outside matches who you are on the inside."*

Alan Cohen

# Chapter Four: Your Feelings

People say, "Trust your feelings." However, you really *can't* trust your feelings because your feelings can change with your thoughts in a millisecond! In this chapter you will:

- Learn how to tell the difference between a feeling and a thought.
- Learn why emotional eating has been such a successful tactic to protect you from your feelings.
- Learn how to experience these feelings.
- Learn how to change your feelings simply by changing your thoughts.

But first, a quick review. Remember these basics: the first step to having the body and health you desire is to visualize yourself actively living in your healthy body. Nothing has a greater ability to alter your physical reality than your thoughts and visualizations. In fact, psychology, philosophy and religion all agree that what you experience in your life is really a product of your individual thoughts. Cognitive therapists have known for decades that *what you think and what you say to yourself has more impact on your mood than the actual circumstances that occur in your life*[vi]. It was fascinating for me to learn in graduate school that for most of us, the circumstances in our lives, for example: poverty, illness and divorce, don't actually cause depression. Our thinking – how we interpret what has happened to us – is the true cause.

Philosophers agree mood is related to thought. Ralph Waldo Emerson stated: "The measure of mental health is the disposition to find good everywhere." Abraham Lincoln said: "Most people are about as happy as they make up their minds to be."[vii] Ernest Holmes writes, "What we outwardly are and what we are to become depends upon what we are thinking."[viii] We hear this same message from many influential people throughout time. Even Jesus Christ taught, "As a man thinks in his heart, so he is."

In the newest research, chemists and neuroscientists have discovered that the mere act of thought alters the balance of your brain chemistry, which can increase your desire to eat. The good news is that there *is* an alternative to overeating. You can alter your lifestyle to more effectively deal with life stresses.

You can find alternative ways to deal with the negative feelings you experience and you can learn to experience feelings without relying on excessive eating or by seeking other chemical relief.

In fact, most people who are overweight are overweight because they eat for emotional reasons rather than for hunger. *Since our human brains are chemically wired for survival and eating is crucial to survival, the brain rewards us with "feel good" brain chemicals when we eat*. This can lead you to overeat when you are stressed. Your brain rewards you with an increase in a "feel good" chemical called serotonin. The brain is truly suited to help you survive in a primitive world where the stresses of danger, hunger, and the elements create chemical reactions. As you become stressed, cortisol and adrenaline levels increase in what is known as *the fight or flight response*. But now, the incessant ringing of the cell phone, incoming text messages and seemingly never-ending demands increase the same chemicals, and you can find yourself fearing for your life when they all happen simultaneously! These unending demands on your time, and the increased fight-or-flight chemicals, can cause you to self-medicate with overeating.

Cortisol and adrenaline are two hormones that increase with stress, especially with fear. They are critically important chemicals for your survival as they initiate the fight or flight response, which helps your body to react quickly to evade danger. When you fight or flee, the physical activity works the cortisol and adrenaline out of your system, bringing you back to calmness. The problem for many of us is that we now live with chronic mental stress and our brains cannot differentiate between actual physical danger and being mentally overwhelmed. To counter the effects and reduce the feelings of stress, many people turn to self-medicating with food, alcohol, drugs, shopping and other addictions, which provide only temporary relief at best. High levels of stress hormones can lead to obesity, addiction and physical illness. A few healthier solutions include: physical exercise, meditation, yoga and deep breathing. For more ideas refer to Chapter 5 and the activities listed under "**Feel Good Chemicals**."

For humans, sedating our feelings with food was a strategy that worked well in the primitive world when we needed to eat large amounts for survival. It does not work today when there's a fast-food restaurant or convenience store on every corner. Despite the lack of physical dangers, our brains erroneously call out for food. In fact, there are chemicals in our brains that cause us to search for food. *Given our complex and overwhelming lifestyles, is it any wonder that we so frequently reach for a dose of serotonin brought about by consuming a tasty food item?*

Let's take a look at serotonin and a few other brain chemicals. These chemicals are called neurotransmitters because they deliver (transmit) messages to the brain (neuro), telling the brain how much hunger to experience, what emotion to feel, when to feel peaceful and when to go into fight or flight mode. In other words, we are wired to receive primitive brain, survival-oriented communication. There are over a hundred known neurotransmitters[ix]. We will focus on a few primary neurotransmitters that are related to food cravings and mood.

Dopamine is pleasure seeking and search initiating, and rewards you with a dose of feel-good serotonin once the search is accomplished. A negative suggestion to yourself about your weight or thinking about your favorite foods can increase the dopamine, which sets up the search and the resulting binge. The overeating creates an increase in serotonin, which brings about a calm, peaceful feeling and puts an end to the binge. Serotonin puts the brakes on how much you eat and decreases your appetite. It also calms you and helps you feel good. Endorphins are natural opiate-like chemicals that cause a state of euphoria as well as a sense of well-being. When your endorphin level is high, you feel safe, loved and see everything as beautiful. Endorphins go up when you eat things you enjoy, participate in cardio-vascular exercise or experience pleasurable activities.

All brain chemicals are influenced by what you think (including what you say to yourself), the activities you are involved in and the foods you eat. The journal activities and *"change your thinking"* activities in this book are designed to increase the serotonin and endorphin levels in your brain to help you feel good and gain control of your eating. If you eat for emotional reasons, it makes perfect sense to eat everything you can. It is part of your subconscious survival, "make it through another day" program.

Fortunately there is a better, healthier and easier lifestyle. This can be accomplished through feeling your feelings. *You don't have to kill your feelings with food and in the process kill yourself.* You can just learn to be aware of and appreciate your feelings. It's good that you used food to survive; survival is imperative. Now the task is to teach your subconscious mind that there is a better way than ingesting chemicals to find good feelings in your world.

**Let's discover the difference between feelings and thoughts:**

| Feelings Are: | Thoughts Are: |
|---|---|
| 1. Associated with sensations in your body. | 1. In your mind. |
| 2. Physical sensations. | 2. Not experienced in your body. |
| 3. Emotions. | 3. Usually evaluations or judgments. |
| 4. Able to be communicated in one word. | 4. Usually expressed in sentences. |

There are three things you can do with a feeling. You can:

- Suppress it.
- Act it out.
- Feel it.

Your feelings are created by your thoughts. Your thoughts actually cause the release of chemicals that create your feelings. Feelings are automatically generated and survival oriented. For example: you're threatened – you feel fear. You automatically know when to run or fight. You don't live in the jungle or on a savannah anymore, but your brain, as a machine, doesn't know that. Can you imagine what would happen if your boss dropped a pile of files on top of the 800 you're already working on and then in self-defense, you stood up and punched him out, then ran from the building screaming? This could have a negative impact on your performance evaluation! If you ignore the physical sensation (fight or flight response) you may decide to eat a large lunch, or go get a self-soothing snack. Food, you have likely learned, can alter your brain chemistry and keep you at a mental functioning baseline.

There are more successful ways to deal with your feelings. *You can learn to feel them rather than suppress them or act them out.* Here are some important factors about feelings that are helpful to know before you practice how to feel. *Feelings do not last forever.* It is your interference and resistance to experience the feelings that lock them in place and do not allow your feelings to change. What you resist persists... ALWAYS!

When you allow yourself to feel a feeling – a sensation in your body – it will usually go away in a few minutes or less. That's less time than it takes to run to the store or to a fast-food restaurant. You just have to be brave the first couple of times you set out to feel. After that, it will be easier because your conscious mind will know you can survive experiencing your feelings. Then doing so will become part of your self-image, which is as you will recall, a subconscious activity.

With the understanding that you can actually change your subconscious mind by exercising your courage to feel, let's get started practicing feeling your feelings. Remember, the attributes of a feeling are felt in the body and can be expressed in one word, which would be either a sensation (such as warm, itchy, tingly, tight, breathless) or an emotion (happy, sad, angry, frustrated, frightened). I bet that you usually have no problem experiencing your pleasant emotions; it's the negative ones that give you problems. So let's practice feeling a feeling, a sensation in the body. This is an exercise that works wonders for all physical sensations including headaches and any stress-related pains.

When you experience anger, sadness, frustration or embarrassment, try this exercise and note how you feel afterward. Notice that every emotion has a physical sensation. Experiencing a feeling means feeling the entire sensation. Fully feeling the sensation allows the feeling to be experienced and then released. *Feeling* takes your mind off the thought that created the sensation, which brings you back to feeling good once again.

## Notes/Journaling

_____

_____

_____

_____

_____

_____

_____

_____

_____

_____

*"Have patience with all things, but first of all, with yourself."*

William James

## Feeling My Feelings Worksheet

Describe the feeling (really look at it; feel it; observe it):

1. Describe the temperature, the size, color, and shape of the feeling. How warm is it? Is it the size of a grape or a plum or a marble? Is it a bright color? Is it a dull color? Which color?

   _____
   _____
   _____
   _____

2. Does it contain liquid? How much does it contain? What is the shape of the container? What kind of liquid does it contain? Is it hot or cold? What is the liquid's consistency?

   _____
   _____
   _____
   _____

3. How big is it now? What shape is it now?

   _____
   _____
   _____
   _____

4. What is its consistency? Really look at the feeling and experience it. Describe it now – start from the top. Keep looking at the feeling. Don't evaluate your thoughts or get into story. No judgment allowed here. Just feel and note in detail what you're feeling now.

   _____
   _____
   _____
   _____

Note how quickly the feeling changes, *how its basic nature is to change and dissipate*. Your feelings are created by chemicals, which are triggered by thought. Feelings can change in milliseconds if you go along with them instead of resist them. As you turn your awareness to the sensation and away from the thought that preceded it, the sensation is guaranteed to change. You will <u>feel</u> better than you felt before. When you feel the feeling rather than responding to it, it simply goes away. Like so many people, you've likely gotten stuck thinking you needed to experience the thought over and over to work through the problem. Your body will actually respond best to the idea of changing the thought and feeling the feeling.

**Remember these three things about feelings:**

1. They are a response to your thoughts.
2. They support your survival by inspiring you to a survival action/reaction.
3. Any overeating you have done to cope with emotions was about survival.

As you learn healthier coping strategies, your eating habits will change. *Don't allow yourself to feel guilty for past overeating*. It helped you survive, and survival is a good thing! What has probably thrown you off balance is a lack of understanding that your primitively developed feelings are not based on current reality. The times and circumstances in which we now live require the conscious selection of different reactions.

To help you make healthier, feeling choices on an ongoing basis, there are two exercises in this chapter to help you. The one we just completed is about "**Feeling Your Feelings**." The second exercise (found at the end of the chapter) is a journaling tool "**Change My Feelings**" using visualization to help you consciously change your feelings by changing your thoughts. This is an adapted tool from the book *Feeling Good* by Dr. David Burns, M.D. Dr. Burn's philosophy is compatible with the thinking of Ernest Holmes: change your thinking, change your life.

The quickest way to change a feeling is to change a thought. Since you now know that feelings are caused by thoughts and you can only think one thought at a time, it follows that your changed thought will generate a new feeling. The journaling and visualization tool will enable you to make rapid changes in your life. It allows you to "redo" every emotional upset and stress during the day, figure out how you would handle it by changing the way you think. Then you visualize the new, better-handled situation. Your subconscious mind will store this new image, and in a surprisingly short period of time, you will find yourself easily and naturally reacting in the way you've been journaling and visualizing! It will seem like magic, but it's not! It's your subconscious mind responding to the new visualization that you consciously chose! You must *want* to change the stressful thought and alter the negative feeling to one that supports a more joyous and fulfilled you. If you believe you deserve to be angry because "that crazy, stupid so and so done you wrong," expect your cortisol level to go up and your food searching behavior to go up with it. You can be justified and right *or* you can be happy, healthy and thin. Which will you choose?

With anger and any other stressful emotion, your cortisol level goes up. When you don't rid yourself of it through fight or flight, you may find yourself trying to manage the anxious feeling it produces by overeating or self-medicating in other ways. The better alternative is to experience the feeling and move on to visualize a healthier, more realistic reaction the next time. Practice the two techniques in this chapter for at least 21[1x] days and note the changes that occur. To incorporate new lifestyle activities into your life, choose one activity from this chapter to practice daily.

**Choose one from the following:**

- Identify and fully experience at least one feeling each day. "**Feeling My Feelings**"
- Complete the "**Changing My Feelings**" entry in your journal each day.

Once you become comfortable with one exercise, add the second one. This will strengthen your mood enhancing skills. Turn to "**My Commitment to Thinking Thin and Healthy**" and date the one exercise you will commit to incorporate into your lifestyle.

---

[1]Psychologists estimate that it takes at least 21 days to form a habit.

(Example)
# Changing My Feelings

Situation (what happened):

*I was at the grocery store and a lady cut right in front of me in line.*

What I said to myself about the situation:

*How dare she do that!*

Feeling (how I felt):

*Angry!!!*

Desire to eat (rate on a 0-10 scale. 1 = no desire, 10 = strong desire):

*A "9"*

How I responded (include: What you said and how you reacted. Did you eat emotionally?):

*I held my anger inside and when I got in the car, I drove to a fast-food restaurant and ordered unhealthy food. I noticed I was still angry.*

How I would like to have handled the situation:

*I would have been calmer, and taken a deep breath or two to relax. I wouldn't have judged her, but would have calmly stated I was in line in front of her, and asked her to go to the back of the line.*

Visualize and feel myself handling the situation this way:

*I see myself calmly, peacefully handling the situation. She is not able to influence my actions.*

## Changing My Feelings Worksheet

Situation (what happened):
_____
_____

What I said to myself about the situation:
_____
_____

Feeling (how I felt):
_____

Desire to eat (rate on a 0-10 scale. 1 = no desire, 10 = strong desire):
_____

How I responded (Include what you said and how you reacted. Did you eat emotionally?):
_____
_____
_____

How I would like to have handled the situation:
_____
_____
_____

Visualize and feel myself handling the situation this way:
_____
_____

# Notes/Journaling

## Notes/Journaling

*"You've braver than you believe, and stronger than you seem, and smarter than you think."*

AA Milne

# Chapter Five: What You Focus On

There is a simple, yet profound skill that can change your life through your thoughts. It is basically learning to keep your eye on the ball. The job of the conscious mind is to identify your goals and set the direction of attaining them in motion. The more time you invest in seeing yourself being and doing the things you desire – such as being slim and eating nutritiously – the faster the message is picked up by the subconscious mind. Then the change in your body and in your behavior becomes automatic.

Remember, the subconscious mind is automatic in its action. It is the conscious mind that sets goals, gathers information, concludes and decides. It does not create results. Your will to act and what you decide to do, which are both conscious acts, do not cause the manifestation of a result. The result is automatic because it is directed by the subconscious mind. Your conscious work is to keep your eye on the goal, to keep your attention focused on what you want versus what you don't want.

It is difficult for most of us to keep our eye on what we want. Most of us have been trained since early childhood to problem-solve – to look for and to find problems that we can solve. Our focus is most frequently on the negative. We are told "no," "don't" and "stop" thousands of times when we are young, and these messages, due to repetition, become more and more powerful in our subconscious minds. The doubt and negative messages get stored in the subconscious and remain there, forever influencing our lives if we let them.

Whenever you think about a goal there are always two possible outcomes. You can get the desired outcome or you can fail to get the desired outcome. If your goal is to be trim and live a healthy lifestyle, you have the possible outcome of being trim and healthy – or not. If you're like most people, when you are thinking about a desired outcome, your focus is on the lack. It makes sense because your focus is on something you don't have. You may say, "but that's the reality, I don't have 'it!'" whether the "it" you don't have is thinness, abundance, relationship or anything else.

When you focus on what you *don't* have, many things happen: first disappointment, then frustration and finally, loss. A whole host of negative emotions arise, and once negativity is let in the door, your thoughts of negativity tend to spiral upward. Everything you think and feel about your body influences your health, vitality and weight. It's your job to nourish and mentally support your ideal weight and health. Let's take a minute to look at the negative or positive self-talk that can influence the outcome.

A simple thought: "I want to be thinner." Sounds positive, doesn't it? Let's look at the words a bit more carefully. "I want to be thinner." makes reference to the fact "I am not thin enough." which could lead to the thought, "In fact, I'm 20 pounds heavier than I want to be." You might justify this thought: "I'm telling myself a FACT!" Your next thought may be, "I'm going to that party, and I have nothing to wear. I'll look terrible in anything I wear. Maybe I won't go. It will be embarrassing to be seen." And on and on and on! Your negative thoughts escalated from a very small negative thought, "I want to be thinner." to a large negative thought, "It will be embarrassing to be seen."

Now let's explore another way of thinking. You could escalate in a positive direction. If you can spiral negatively, you can do the same positively. Even if your weight is really an issue for you, you can always find small things about your body or your choices to feel good about. For example, starting with a small thought, "Wow! I remembered to eat a healthy breakfast this morning." escalates to "I love the healthy food choices I make, they make me feel good." "I feel energetic and strong." "I know my body will really respond to this new habit." A small positive "Wow! I ate a healthy breakfast." started the journey to the joyous expectancy of positive results!

Remember, you have absolute control over what you say to yourself because your choices, evaluations and judgments are all conscious activities and you are in the driver's seat where they are concerned. Every statement of desire has an equal possibility of missing the mark or of attaining your desire. Let's look at some of the statements you can make about your body. See if they are bringing you closer or taking you further away from your desired outcome.

| **Focus On Positive** | **Focus On Negative** |
|---|---|
| • I am so proud of the food choices I am making. | • I've been dieting all week and haven't lost a pound. |
| • My body is healthy and radiant. | • I don't want to be fat anymore (focus on fat). |
| • I am health and well-being. | • This outfit makes me look fat. |
| • I am the out picturing of my every thought. | • I can't _____ until I'm thinner (implies I'm not thin enough). |
| • I know I can accomplish everything I desire by keeping my focus on it. | • I want to be thinner. |

Take a moment and review your self-talk and be honest with yourself. *Have you been focusing on what you want or what you don't want?* You get what you focus on, whether it's the desired outcome or the lack of it. This is the Law of Attraction and it *always* works!

**Love Your Body**

An easy and empowering way to maintain your focus on what you want versus what you don't want is to acknowledge the things about yourself that you like and feel good about. Pay attention to them and keep your focus on them. Even if you are currently overweight, I am sure there are still many things you enjoy about your body. There are aspects of it that bring you pleasure. Perhaps it's your hair, your nails, your ability to walk, your soft skin or your expressive eyes. When you look in the mirror, focus on those positive aspects and develop the habit of listing at least three positive qualities about your body each day.

The worksheet that follows is a place for you to keep a daily record of three qualities of your body that you are happy with. Keeping your focus on the positive will always help you attain your desires. It's okay to repeat some of the aspects you like. View each day as a brand-new day!

*"If you could only love enough, you could be the most powerful person in the world."*

Emmet Fox

*Thinking Thin Through Spiritual and Mental Steps*

# Things I Love About My Body Worksheet

On the worksheet below, write three things each day that you like/love about your body.

Sunday:
1. _____
2. _____
3. _____

Monday
1. _____
2. _____
3. _____

Tuesday
1. _____
2. _____
3. _____

Wednesday
1. _____
2. _____
3. _____

Thursday
1. _____
2. _____
3. _____

Friday
1. _____
2. _____
3. _____

Saturday
1. _____
2. _____
3. _____

Have you ever noticed how wonderfully your day goes when you wake up excited, energetic and looking forward to every moment? It is because you manifest not only with your words, but with your words accompanied with your feelings. When you are excited and happy, everything comes up roses. Unfortunately, the opposite is also true of negative feelings. In understanding emotions and how all this works, you can simplify the process by noting that the feelings you experience can be broken down into two simple categories:

**One Category feels *Good*. The other Category feels *Bad*.**

Recognize two things about these states of feeling. First of all, all feelings can be useful for you. They are actually your aides, or guides if you will, to tell you if you are on track to meeting your goal[xi]. As goal-striving beings, when your behavior and thoughts have you on track to meet your goals, you feel good. When you are off track, you feel bad. All feelings can be used as a barometer of how "on track" you are by what you are saying and doing. If you're feeling badly, look at your behavior or thoughts. You will most likely realize that you are doing something that is not supporting your desired outcome. The following worksheet is a four-step exercise to assist you in focusing on what you truly want, rather than eating to numb your feelings.

## Notes/Journaling

_____
_____
_____
_____
_____
_____
_____
_____
_____
_____

*Thinking Thin Through Spiritual and Mental Steps*

# What I Want Worksheet

1. Note what you are thinking or doing. Is it moving you toward your goal? (For example, I am at the grocery store buying cookies for a snack.)

　_____

　_____

　_____

　_____

2. Identify what you truly want. (For example: I want to be thin.)

　_____

　_____

　_____

　_____

3. Visualize yourself having what you want. (For example: I spend a few seconds seeing myself at my ideal body weight.)

　_____

　_____

　_____

　_____

4. Take one small step toward its accomplishment. (For example: I put the cookies down and move to the produce department where I buy an apple instead.)

　_____

　_____

　_____

　_____

Note the words "small step" in the previous exercise. A small step will change the direction of your focus and get you back on track. Also remember the concept of negativity or great positive expectancy started with one small thought. The spiral of negativity is how low self-esteem or an eating binge starts. *Turn that spiral in the opposite direction and you get improved self-esteem and healthy eating habits.* The simple act of thinking one small thought in a positive or negative direction will turn it all around. It's a process, but the direction you start spiraling in will take on its own synergy.

Lynn Grabhorn, in her book *Excuse Me, Your Life is Waiting* refers to changing your thoughts as "flip switching." To help in behavioral changes, the sooner you can flip from one thought to another, the better. It's easier to flip from the small thought "I want to be thinner." versus waiting until you go all the way down to being embarrassed about your body. But wherever you notice the negativity and as soon as you notice it, that is the time to start. *You can "flip switch" a mood by focusing on the desired outcome or on things that make you happy, or by doing something that makes you really happy!*

In Chapter Four, we looked at chemicals that can alter your mood. Now let's look at activities that increase serotonin and endorphins in the body. Remember, serotonin puts the brakes on your appetite, calms you and helps you feel safe. Endorphins make you feel happy and content. In order to live in absolute health, both mentally and physically, and be able to control your eating, you need to have a healthy balance of brain chemicals. Let's look at a list of activities that affect serotonin and endorphin production and what you can do to change your mood to magnetize more health to you.

## Notes/Journaling

_____

_____

_____

_____

_____

_____

_____

*Thinking Thin Through Spiritual and Mental Steps*

| **Endorphins** | **Serotonin** |
|---|---|

- Being in love.
- Enjoying the company of others.
- Eating foods you enjoy.
- Any pleasurable experience.
- Connecting with nature.
- Laughing.
- Singing.
- All physical exercise, especially cardiovascular such as jogging, walking, swimming, biking.

- Calming thoughts.
- Meditation or yoga.
- Deep breathing.
- Gardening.
- Listening to music.
- Floating in a pool.
- Walking by water.
- Eating certain foods, especially bananas, papayas, passion fruit and pineapple.

In the space provided below, add your personal favorite activities to each list. Things that bring you joy and excitement go on the endorphin side. Things you do that help you feel calm and relaxed go on the serotonin side.

**Endorphins**                                  **Serotonin**

_____          _____

_____          _____

_____          _____

_____          _____

_____          _____

_____          _____

We will now add two more powerful tools to your tool chest. The more tools you have and master, the greater ability you will have to feel good and control negative thinking. The first tool is "flip switching" and getting happy. Lynn Grabhorn refers to this as "getting jazzed." All of us have a repertoire of things that can change our mood by simply doing them. As shown on the previous list, running, swimming, singing and listening to music are all activities that can increase our serotonin and/or endorphin levels. There are also things you *think* about that have the power to change your mood and brain chemistry just by *remembering them*. I know that when you look for them, you'll find you have memories of events or experiences that bring you great joy. Some examples could be:

- The birth of a child.

- The first time you saw your grandchild.

- A favorite place you visit.

- A friend who always lifts your spirits.

- A movie you love .

- Think of something someone said that made you feel wonderful. (For me, it's an old boyfriend of mine who told me, "You're not beautiful, you're gorgeous…You're not smart, you're brilliant…You're not funny, you're hysterical…" It lifts my self-esteem and brings me joy every time I think of it, so I think of it often!).

To help you keep your focus on joyous experiences and positive events, the following worksheet is designed to help you recall past positive experiences.

## My Joy Journal

Memories or experiences that fill your heart with joy.

- _____
- _____
- _____

Places you've been that made you happy.

- _____
- _____
- _____

Movies that bring you joy.

- _____
- _____
- _____

Songs or plays that make you smile or laugh.

- _____
- _____
- _____

Things you or others have said or done that make you laugh.

- _____
- _____
- _____

Things that give you pride in yourself or others.

- _____
- _____
- _____

Your goal should be to live your life on a physical and mental plane that supports you in feeling good always. Feeling good is your natural state. Your body and mind – the chemicals in your brain – are all designed to keep you in balance, which is feeling good! Ultimately, you have absolute control over your thoughts, interpretations and how you choose to feel. Turn to "**My Commitment to Thinking Thin and Healthy**" worksheet and mark the date you commit to the practices in this chapter. These tools will put you back in the driver's seat toward emotional balance, which feels very, very good!

## Notes/Journaling

_____
_____
_____
_____
_____
_____
_____
_____
_____
_____
_____
_____
_____
_____
_____
_____
_____
_____

## Notes/Journaling

*"Health is a start of complete harmony of the body, mind and spirit. When one is free from physical disabilities and mental distractions, the gates of the soul open."*

B.K.S. Iyengar

# Chapter Six: Change

This chapter's focus is on change. We have all heard that change is the one constant in life. Given that we know change is inevitable, why do we resist it and why is it so difficult and painful?

Whenever I read or write, I keep a dictionary near me. "Change" has ten different definitions, but one of the best definitions is:

"to put or take (a thing) in place of something else; to substitute: as he changed his clothes."

The definition is perfect and also defines our plan of the day with this program. The goal is to replace a self-defeating behavior with a healthy, self-enhancing behavior. You've learned in previous chapters anything you focus on persists. Therefore, if your goal is to lose weight and you focus on your weight or your need to lose weight (which really is a focus on being overweight) your weight will likely increase. I know from personal experience that the times I gained the most weight were the times I was thinking about dieting the most. The subconscious mind, fearing a shortage of food, will guide you to say yes to all the food you encounter. I've heard before that D.I.E.T. stands for **D**ine **I**n **E**xcess **T**omorrow!

In this chapter we look at a structured yet simple way you can substitute a self-enhancing and positive eating pattern for a self-defeating and destructive one. This lifestyle skill will help you attain your ideal weight, energy and your healthiest body yet! Change has been studied a fair amount, which is a good thing since it is life's one constant! Here are some keys to remember about change and human personality:

- For change to occur in the material/physical world your mental image must be the first to change. You must *believe* that you have something before you can achieve it. This is true for your body as well as for anything else in your life. It will only be done when you believe.

- Joseph Murphy said, "We are all creatures of habit—habit is a function of our subconscious mind. We learned to swim, ride a bicycle, dance and drive a car by consciously doing these things over and over again until they established tracks in our subconscious mind. Then, the automatic habit action of the subconscious mind took over.[xii]" You have absolute power to change your habit patterns. It makes sense that if you develop these automatic patterns through repetition of a consciously chosen activity, you can once again consciously choose a new activity and develop a new pattern.

- One of my favorite books on personality and change is *Psycho-Cybernetics* by Maxwell Maltz, MD, FICS. Dr. Maltz states that any mental image held in thought will become your new self-identity. He suggests that you reserve your judgment for twenty-one days, as self-image change takes twenty-one days (average) of active practice. Once the new image is accepted by your subconscious mind, the change will be automatic.

- Your biochemistry is rigged to draw you toward actions and activities that help make you feel good. You can even alter the feel-good brain chemicals by your thoughts. All of your survival instincts lead you to a combination of brain chemicals that leave you feeling satisfied, happy, and even ecstatic! Therefore, as you look for new habits to replace the old, you need to look for activities that lift your spirits.

In order to create change, you must first take stock of your goals and where you want to go. When you plan a trip you need to know where you are and the location of your final destination. With these two facts you can develop a plan to reach your goal.

To eliminate self-defeating behavior:

1. Set goals. If you attempt to make a change without knowing clearly where you want to go, it is easy to get off track. (For example: I want to be a healthy weight with energy to do all I desire!)

2. Identify the behavior that is in your way of accomplishing the goal (such as overeating – especially sweets). Develop a "**Cost/Benefit Worksheet**" (the worksheet and an example are provided later in this chapter) to increase awareness of the damaging effects of the behavior and increase motivation for change.

3. Identify alternate self-enhancing behaviors. These would be behaviors that bring you the rewards and pleasures that you received from the benefit side of the "**Cost/Benefit Worksheet**." For example, the benefits of overeating are "it relaxes me," "it tastes good," or "it's social." A healthy alternative for "it relaxes me" could be deep breathing or a warm bath.

As you begin your change of lifestyle journey, take a moment to evaluate where you are right now, and where you'd like to go in relation to your body. You'll be setting goals for all areas of your life in the next chapter. Complete the following worksheet, being truthful about your current physical state and specific about your desired goal.

## Notes/Journaling

*"Your life does not get better by chance, it gets better by change."*

Jim Rohn

## My Physical State Worksheet

**My Health**

Now: _____

_____

Goal: _____

_____

**My Energy**

Now: _____

_____

Goal: _____

_____

**My Weight**

Now: _____

_____

Goal: _____

_____

**My Body Shape**

Now: _____

_____

Goal: _____

_____

**How I Feel in My Clothes**

Now: _____

_____

Goal: _____

_____

**My Thoughts about My Body**

Now: _____

_____

Goal: _____

_____

Knowing where you are and where you want to be will help you make commitments that support your desired outcome. Motivation is frequently born out of the disparity of where you are and the dream of where you want to be. Changing your self-defeating behaviors into self-enhancing ones can be done with greater ease if you have a substitute activity – or in Webster's words, you need "to put or take (a thing) in place of something else." The reason you fall into self-destructive habits is because of the "rewards" they bring you. For example, with overeating, you may feel relaxed and the food tastes good. These aren't actually long-term rewards, though. They have long-term negative consequences. Identifying healthy alternative habits that bring you rewards that are self-enhancing in the long-term (for example: choosing food that tastes great and is low-calorie) is essential in making a lifestyle change.

The following journal exercise will provide a very specific and clear message to your subconscious mind about the importance and benefit of accepting change. The amazing fact about the **Cost/Benefit Worksheet** is that the consequences of the behaviors, listed on the cost side, are *always* higher. How do I know this in advance? If the benefits outweigh the costs, the behavior is self-enhancing and wouldn't be problematic and require a change. It wouldn't cause the problem you desire to overcome. Let's take a look at the behavior of overeating and come up with a list of Cost-versus-Benefit.

## Notes/Journaling

_____
_____
_____
_____
_____
_____
_____
_____

*Thinking Thin Through Spiritual and Mental Steps*

(Example)

## Cost/Benefit

<u>Overeating – especially sugary snacks</u>
*List the behavior (habit) you want to change.*

**Costs**                                    **Benefits**

I gain weight.                    It relaxes me.

It zaps my energy.             It tastes good.

It's unhealthy.                  It's social.

My clothes don't fit.

I don't look as attractive.

It's expensive.

My self-esteem plummets.

*"Sorry, there's no magic bullet. You gotta eat healthy and live healthy to be healthy and look healthy. End of story!"*

Morgan Spurlock

*Thinking Thin Through Spiritual and Mental Steps*

# Cost/Benefit Worksheet

*List the behavior (habit) you want to change.*

**Costs**                                    **Benefits**

Initiating change in a habit can bring up fear because you are unsure of the consequences. To change a habitual pattern feels like a risk. The biggest problem is, if you don't risk the change, you are guaranteed to stay the same. In the case of self-defeating behaviors, there will always be a negative cost associated with staying the same.

One great way of working toward eliminating self-defeating behaviors is to have a ready plan of "alternative behaviors" that can be substituted. It is critical in making changes that you don't leave yourself without alternative behaviors to fall back on. It is always easier to make changes when you have a plan in place. If you plan now, you won't feel stranded when temptation hits.

On the next page is a worksheet titled "**My Dozen Alternative Behaviors List**," where you can plan up to a dozen self-enhancing activities as a substitute for the self-defeating behavior of overeating. This list works hand-in-hand with the **Cost/Benefit Worksheet**. For example: for the benefit of "it relaxes me," you could list as alternatives taking a bubble bath, going for a walk, or listening to music. For the benefit of "it tastes good" you could drink some sparkling water, have some fresh fruit, or chew sugar-free gum.

## Notes/Journaling

_____

_____

_____

_____

_____

_____

_____

_____

_____

_____

*Thinking Thin Through Spiritual and Mental Steps*
# My Dozen Alternative Behaviors List

_____

*A Self-Defeating Behavior I'd Like to Eliminate*

**List twelve healthy alternative behaviors: (i.e. deep breathing, a warm bath)**

1. _____

2. _____

3. _____

4. _____

5. _____

6. _____

7. _____

8. _____

9. _____

10. _____

11. _____

12. _____

I hope you find all the tools and worksheets in this chapter helpful. My greatest desire is to support you in making positive changes to live in optimal health and increased happiness. Once you have completed the "**My Physical State Worksheet**," "**Cost/Benefit Worksheet**" and "**My Dozen Alternative Behaviors Worksheet**," review them often to maintain motivation. Keep the "**My Dozen Alternative Behaviors**" worksheet with you and choose healthy behaviors versus the ones that are self-defeating. Fill in the "**My Commitment to Thinking Thin and Healthy**" worksheet at the beginning of this book. Being prepared and working in mind, as well as making behavioral changes, will always lead you to your desired outcome.

## Notes/Journaling

_____
_____
_____
_____
_____
_____
_____
_____
_____
_____
_____
_____
_____
_____
_____
_____
_____
_____

**Notes/Journaling**

*"If you do what you've always done, you'll get what you've always gotten."*

Tony Robbins

# Chapter Seven: Are You Smushed?

Your desire to make changes can seem overwhelming at times. Making one simple change a week can add up to a hefty lifestyle change over a matter of time. You are not as imperfect as you think. We are all perfect images of God, and by simply fine tuning a few mental skills and practicing them, you can come closer to realizing your perfection. Remember that before a change can occur in your manifest world, it must originate in your mind. By simply focusing on one change at a time, and sticking with it daily until it becomes second nature, you will eventually develop all the skills required to become slim and maintain slimness with natural, intuitive ease!

**You Eat How You Live**

Is your life cool, calm and filled with abundance in all areas? Does your life flow with grace and ease? Or do you find yourself smushed between work, family and social demands with little time to reflect, pray and live in the moment? Most of us live in a very hectic reality. Your expectations of material accomplishment and continually increasing expectations of success can put major stress on your life. The term "smushed," which I define as "the elimination of time and space due to the taking in and taking on of everything" is a word that describes many of our lives.

I found through the years that it is critical to frequently go through my life and identify the time wasters and even pick out some of the wonderfully important things I do that don't contribute to my goals. This helps me to eliminate some activities from my life and pinpoint other activities where I should simply say "no." You need to keep your calendar reasonable, with time to breathe deeply and meditate so you don't become smushed! For your health and well-being, balance is absolutely necessary. A life overly filled with service, work and chores leaves no room for movement and no time for creativity; you need time to reflect, to be in the moment and love your family and friends. Being smushed takes away all the joy of the moment. Life is <u>way</u> more than just a to-do list!

To get your life back on track and headed in the direction you desire requires some reflection and that's what you'll spend time doing now. The following exercises are designed to:

- Help you identify your values.

- Identify your goals so you will develop clarity about where you want to go based on your values.

- Identify how you spend your time so you will be able to assess if the way you spend your time is helping you reach your goals.

- Make changes in your time schedule as needed to ensure that your priorities are being given attention.

You'll have worksheets along the way to help you make the process fun and keep it structured.

The first exercise is to write out your own obituary! Describe how you would like to be remembered. You can include facts about your family, life, friendships, career, your spiritual development, the values you embraced and the dreams that you cherished. Take time to really reflect on your life. Highlight the aspects of your life that are most important to you. Take time now to complete the exercise because it will help you identify your values.

## **Notes/Journaling**

_____
_____
_____
_____
_____
_____
_____
_____
_____

*Thinking Thin Through Spiritual and Mental Steps*

# The Obituary for:

Good job on completing your desired obituary. You might have learned things you would like to change about yourself or your lifestyle. Remember how important it is to feel good about yourself? It is easy to forget how accomplished you actually are and to focus on what you *don't* have. This next exercise will focus on your accomplishments in various areas of life. Use the worksheets that follow to list all the accomplishments you have, big *and* small. On my list of accomplishments, I even included my life-saving certificate I earned as a teenager! It was a significant accomplishment for me then and it still is. Nothing is too small!

## Notes/Journaling

## My Accomplishments

**Spiritual:**

_____

_____

_____

_____

_____

_____

_____

_____

_____

**Physical:**

_____

_____

_____

_____

_____

_____

_____

_____

_____

# My Accomplishments

**Family:**

_____

_____

_____

_____

_____

_____

_____

_____

_____

**Career:**

_____

_____

_____

_____

_____

_____

_____

_____

_____

## My Accomplishments

**Social:**

_____

_____

_____

_____

_____

_____

**Financial:**

_____

_____

_____

_____

_____

_____

**Intellectual:**

_____

_____

_____

_____

_____

_____

Keep these worksheets and continue to add to them over the years. They are a place to record all the successful moments you have. Add additional accomplishments as you manifest them and review them frequently. Doing so increases your endorphin level. You will feel better and be in better control of your eating and your mood. The accomplishments of your past are the foundation upon which you can build your future. When you feel the power of your accomplishments, they will help you move forward with ever-increasing ease.

Let's take some time now to look at your current goals. Think about the goals you have for the near future and those in the far-off distance. A big part of getting un-smushed is to recognize that in your lifetime you can focus on your goals and desires of today, while having dreams for the future. As time and energy become freed up, you can take some dreams off your long-term goal list and put them on your to-do list! Getting ideas, dreams and goals on paper and continually adding to them is a responsible first step toward their completion. Goal setting *always* starts with writing down your goals.

So, set yourself up for some major success by writing down all of your goals. On the following worksheets write down all the goals you have for your life – what would you like to learn? Where would you like to go? What would you like to create? Don't leave any area of your life neglected. Balance is the key to a wonderful life, so make sure you have at least two goals in each category.

## Notes/Journaling

_____
_____
_____
_____
_____
_____
_____
_____
_____

## Goals I Want to Accomplish

**Spiritual:**

_____
_____
_____
_____
_____
_____
_____

**Physical:**

_____
_____
_____
_____
_____
_____
_____

**Family:**

_____
_____
_____
_____
_____
_____
_____

# Goals I Want to Accomplish

**Career:**

_____
_____
_____
_____
_____

**Social:**

_____
_____
_____
_____
_____

**Financial:**

_____
_____
_____
_____
_____

**Intellectual:**

_____
_____
_____
_____
_____

Your focus in getting un-smushed is to identify all the activities you are currently engaged in that don't contribute to your priorities and goals. Identify activities that may feel critical but truly could be better left for someone else to do. In fact, you could be benefiting other people by allowing them the opportunity to experience that activity (for example: be in charge of the church social planning committee) or by paying someone to help you do the chores around the house that you don't enjoy. I have always felt wonderful being able to pay someone to clean my house, fix the car, etc. It is always a win-win situation. Keeping money flowing to those who help us will increase our prosperity consciousness as well as our time consciousness.

The next activity is to help you identify how you spend your time. The following time schedule is blocked out into one-hour increments for the week. List how you spend your time. Write down everything: household chores, work, church activities, hobbies, family time, social time, TV, computer time, reading, and other leisure activities. Take time to complete this schedule and attempt to list every activity. If you don't have a regularly scheduled time to do chores such as laundry or housework just list them somewhere you typically might get them done.

## Notes/Journaling

_____
_____
_____
_____
_____
_____
_____
_____
_____
_____
_____

*"Everything changed the day she figured out there was exactly enough time for the important things in her life."*

Brian Andreas

# My Personal Time Schedule

|        | Sunday | Monday | Tuesday | Wednesday | Thursday | Friday | Saturday |
|--------|--------|--------|---------|-----------|----------|--------|----------|
| 6:00   |        |        |         |           |          |        |          |
| 7:00   |        |        |         |           |          |        |          |
| 8:00   |        |        |         |           |          |        |          |
| 9:00   |        |        |         |           |          |        |          |
| 10:00  |        |        |         |           |          |        |          |
| 11:00  |        |        |         |           |          |        |          |
| 12:00  |        |        |         |           |          |        |          |
| 1:00   |        |        |         |           |          |        |          |
| 2:00   |        |        |         |           |          |        |          |
| 3:00   |        |        |         |           |          |        |          |
| 4:00   |        |        |         |           |          |        |          |
| 5:00   |        |        |         |           |          |        |          |
| 6:00   |        |        |         |           |          |        |          |
| 7:00   |        |        |         |           |          |        |          |
| 8:00   |        |        |         |           |          |        |          |
| 9:00   |        |        |         |           |          |        |          |
| 10:00  |        |        |         |           |          |        |          |

# Notes/Journaling

*Thinking Thin Through Spiritual and Mental Steps*

Once your worksheet is complete, it's time to get to work and compare how you spend your time with your values and goals. You might discover you are on track. Or, you may identify that one of your goals is to relax and discover that you are booked up 24/7. We all have the same 24 hours a day to work with. H. Jackson Brown, Jr. once said, "Don't say you don't have enough time. You have exactly the same number of hours per day that were given to Helen Keller, Pasteur, Michelangelo, Mother Teresa, Leonardo da Vinci, Thomas Jefferson, and Albert Einstein." Living in balance can be a struggle given the demands on your time, even though many of those activities are desirable or even wonderful! You may need to say "no" to some demands if appropriate.

Set up a schedule and follow it through. You frequently need to look at how you're spending your time and eliminate some of the activities you've out grown or that just don't fit with what you desire anymore. I would suggest doing this at least twice a year. Remember, you *can* do it all, just not all right now! A friend of mine once told me "Pam, you don't have to live your whole life this year!" Thank you, Patti, for that great observation! I remember it often and will frequently put things I want, or things I want to do, on my goal list, recognizing that as I focus on and accomplish today's priorities I will be tackling new goals/projects in the future. If your schedule has you running wild, take a good hard look at your goals and see if some of your present projects would best be put off until next spring or next year. It is not defeat to balance your life. It is sane; it makes total sense and may be just what the doctor ordered to get your brain chemistry cooled down and your life de-smushed.

If you put off involvement in activities that make you feel smushed, will that free up time for your involvement in meditation, putzing in the garden or going for a long-promised walk in beautiful nature? Remember, you are benefiting others by allowing them the opportunity to serve and grow when you release over-involvement. Believe it or not, someone capable always steps forward!

If you find that your life is lacking stimulation, you might pull something from your goal list and place it on your daily schedule as a "to do." Again, remember that balance is the key. Most of us will find ourselves swinging between overwhelmed and underwhelmed at different times in our lives. You always have control over how you spend your time, and which priorities you choose to focus on during any given time. Keeping balance will add joy to your life and decrease your overeating, which is related to stress, anxiety, and all the negative feelings you experience when you're overwhelmed. When your schedule is overly full, your dinner plate might tend to be overly full as well. As you clear your calendar, watch your plate clear up too!

De-smushing your life will bring you into peace and harmony with your schedule, so you can live your life in the Now, where you can savor the sweet blessings of each moment. Instead of smushing your schedule with excess activity and your body with excess food in an attempt to feel good, you'll be able to relax in the moment, appreciate what you have and the activity at hand. It takes a little time and some planning to journal, pray and meditate… in other words, to practice the skills in this guidebook. Turn to "**My Commitment to Thinking Thin and Healthy**" and mark the date you commit to this practice. By de-smushing your life, I hope you will find time for all the life-affirming activities in this book. I know they will help guide you to absolute health and the body you visualize.

## Notes/Journaling

_____
_____
_____
_____
_____
_____
_____
_____
_____
_____
_____
_____
_____
_____
_____
_____

## Notes/Journaling

*"Letting go gives us freedom, and freedom is the only condition for happiness."*

Thich Nhat Hanh

# What's Next?

Congratulations on completing the exercises and worksheets in this book! If you've skipped some I strongly encourage you to go back and complete them all. Finding balance in your life is essential for you to lose weight and maintain a healthy lifestyle. The pace of the life you lead might all too frequently lead you to overeat. Willpower has proven to be finite in life. If you are overexerted at work and overwhelmed with obligations, it will be difficult to utilize willpower to change your eating and exercise patterns. The exercises in this book are designed to help you bring spirituality and sound psychological principles into your life. This will help you de-stress and find natural joy and peace, and achieve your weight loss in a natural manner.

Having a like-minded community to support you in your weight loss goals is another powerful way to increase the likelihood of your success. Group support is a powerful step toward success and it's very exciting to share the journey with friends. Such a group exists at PerfectWeightMadeEasy.com. We have weekly blog posts, teleconferences, live classes and private coaching. If you are interested in bringing *Perfect Weight Made Easy* to your church, workplace or organization, contact me for more information.

I thank you for your commitment to health and for sharing this journey with me. I hope you will join the Perfect Weight Made Easy community today, and I look forward to continuing to participate in this journey with you!

# Notes/Journaling

## Notes/Journaling

# Notes/Journaling

## Notes/Journaling

*"In everything give thanks."*

Khalil Gibran

# Acknowledgements

A special thank you to Cliff Edwards. Your guidance and friendship truly can move mountains. The fact that this book is complete proves that!

I want to thank Nancy Conklin, Jim Snelling and Amy Anderson for your editorial support. This manuscript would not be in existence without your talents.

*"Go confidently in the direction of your dreams. Live the life you imagined."*

Henry David Thoreau

# About the Author

Dr. Pamela S. Chapman helps people who struggle with issues of excess weight, unhealthy eating habits, and poor self-image develop the habits and make the choices that lead to vital, energetic health and ideal weight. Pam's interest in both physical and psychological health and weight loss methodologies arise from her personal challenges coping with both issues.

Raised in an abusive family with physical violence and rejection as her earliest foundation, Pam found comfort and acceptance in over eating and substance abuse. Her earliest memory of the relief that over eating offered her was around the age of five or six. Scared and stressed while witnessing a physical fight between her mother and grandmother, Pam made the startling discovery that eating pastries temporarily calmed her mind and helped her feel better.

Over the years her dependency on food as solace grew and led to years of obesity, yo-yo dieting and poor self-esteem. She has experienced first-hand the short-term elation of crash diets with their rapid weight loss and the heartache of having the weight return. Topping the scales at 228 pounds, Pam understands the pain and self-loathing that accompany food addiction and obesity.

Through the support of therapy, coaching, personal study, and self-reflection, Pam eventually discovered a means to cultivate self-esteem, happiness, and health. Using the life-changing techniques of cognitive therapy, visualization with focused feeling, and a balanced exercise and food plan, she found a simple path to life-long nutritious eating and maintaining healthy weight.

The greatest joy that Pam has experienced is sharing her success and helping others to overcome their weight and self-esteem issues through *Your Perfect Weight Made Easy* – a program for weight loss and well-being. Based on lessons from own her life journey, Pam's approach is one of compassion, understanding and personal accountability. She can show you how to add structure and make empowering choices so that you develop new ways of thinking, being, and living. Then she will assist you step by step on your journey to an energetic, joyful and successful future.

Pam is a Licensed Clinical Social Worker (LCSW) with over twenty-five years of helping individuals overcome depression and discover the joy and peace of living free from chemical, food, and other addictions. She was an instructor for seven years at Mira Costa College in Oceanside, CA. teaching classes in Healthy Aging and was the Executive Director of Tierrasanta Village of San Diego for over two years. Through teaching and the village experience, Pam met hundreds of healthy, thriving people and has created numerous seminars on life-long health and vitality.

Pam has a Doctorate in Religious Studies with an emphasis in counseling, a Master's Degree in Social Work, and is a Certified Therapeutic Recreation Specialist. Her other publications include articles on healthy aging, the value of exercise, and the village movement, published in *Caring for the Ages* (a publication of the American Medical Directors Association.)

Pam is a nationally and internationally acclaimed speaker, presenting lively talks to colleges, churches, and other organizations. Her emphasis is always on the art and practice of joyful living and increasing one's health and self-esteem. Through her seminars and speaking engagements, she demonstrates a passion for spiritual practice, physical activity and life balance.

Her insights, experiences and encouraging, supportive message can be read regularly on her blog at http://PerfectWeightMadeEasy.com. Pam frequently teaches and presents via teleconferences and trainings. She is available to speak at your organization on the topics of healthy weight loss, self-esteem, and Aging Magnificently. You can find additional information, inspiration and support, follow Pam's events and correspond with her at: http://YourPerfectWeightMadeEasy.com.

Pam and her husband John currently have their home base in Ogden, Utah. She enjoys travel, writing, and entertaining. After living most of her life near the perpetually sunny, warm beaches of San Diego, she now delights in the wonder and beauty of mountain living with its distinctive seasons and snow.

# End Notes

[i] Ogden, Dr. Cynthia. "Prevalence of Childhood and Adult Obesity in the United States, 2011-2012." *Journal of the American Medical Association*. 311.8: 2014, 806-814.

[ii] Anderson, Dr. Wayne Scott. *Discover Your Optimal Health*. Da Capo Press: Boston, 2013.

[iii] Moynihan, Julie. "Do Diets Work?" *Scientific American Frontiers*. 2014.

[iv] Fox, Kate. "Mirror-Mirror." Social Issues Research Center: 1997.

[v] Braden, Gregg. *The Isaiah Effect*. Three Rivers Press: New York, 2000.

[vi] Burns, Dr. David D. *Feeling Good*. New American Library: New York, 1980. 28.

[vii] Maltz, Dr. Maxwell. *Psycho-Cybernetics*. Prentice-Hall, Englewood Cliffs. 1960. 90-95.

[viii] Holmes, Ernest. *The Science of Mind*. G. P. Putnam's Sons: New York, 1938. 140.

[ix] Paulak, Dr. Laura. *Stop Gaining Weight*. BioMed General: Concord, 2004.

[x] Maltz, Dr. Maxwell. *Psycho-Cybernetics*. Prentice-Hall, Englewood Cliffs. 1960. xxiii.

[xi] Grabhorn, Lynn. *Excuse Me, Your Life is Waiting*. Hampton Roads Publishing: Charlottesville, 2000. 27

[xii] Murphy, Dr. Joseph *The Power of Your Subconscious Mind*. Reward Books: Paramus, 2000. 209-210

Made in the USA
San Bernardino, CA
05 November 2014